ERECTILE DYSFUNCTION

Boost Your Sexual Instinct And Eliminate Performance Anxiety Forever (Sexual Desire, Low Libido, Relationship And Romance)

INTRODUCTION

Erectile dysfunction can be defined as one of the greatest fears of men. Nothing kills the mood faster than trying desperately to get an erection during sex. It has been described as one of the last few great taboos that some men still won't admit to having. It happens to at least one out of ten men. Most times, it is due to insecurities on the man's part or lack of understanding on the woman's part. Statistics has also shown that it leads to the failure of about two in ten marriages of the affected population.

Very few men have the courage to talk about their conditions or even get help. Some go as far as lashing out at their partners and blaming them for their inability to have sex. One man brave enough to speak about his situation was Peter (not his real name), a sixty-year-old salesman, who has a wife and son. Peter became impotent after radiotherapy, while he was undergoing treatment for prostate cancer. He explained how he experienced every man's greatest fear and still managed to pull through. He was no saint; initially, he was frustrated and depressed because the disease left him feeling like he wasn't a whole man. Finding out that you wouldn't be able to make love to your wife again was a major setback. The radiotherapy was meant to kill the cancer cells in his body, but it ended up doing more than that. Peter stated that he would have rather suffered every other side effect of radiotherapy than the one he got. It helped a lot that he had a supportive wife by his side, and together they sought out different specialists to help manage the condition. While he wasn't able to cure his erectile dysfunction, Peter was able to find ways to live with it. Today he has a relatively healthy sex life.

The moral of the story is that; even though the disease will make you feel inadequate and less of a man, there are still ways left to enjoy your sex life. It's not an easy journey, but you just have to believe that things will get better.

As you progress from one chapter to the other, you will see that there is hope nearer than you think. By the time you get to the end of this guide, you will have the knowledge you need to get your sexual life back in action.

CHAPTER ONE
AN OVERVIEW OF ERECTILE DYSFUNCTION

Another name for erectile dysfunction is impotence. Erectile dysfunction or ED as it is often called is a kind of sexual dysfunction that is associated with the inability of men to perform sexually. The penis is usually flaccid, and most times the man cannot get an erection. In some cases, however, when he does get an erection, it will not last for long. The lack of erection is usually a problem during sex. ED is mostly found in older men, but it has been reported to happen to younger people as well. An erect penis is as a result of the hydraulic effect of venous blood flowing into it. The blood is stored in sponge-like tissues within the phallus. During sexual activities, nervous signals are transported from the brain down to the penis causing it to become aroused. The arousal occurs as a result of the increase in blood flow to the penis which then leads to an erection. As soon as the blood is in the penis, it's trapped within the corpora cavernosa due to pressure. As a result of this, the penis expands and holds the erection. The penis goes back to its weak and soft state as soon as the veins open up and the inflow of blood reduces.

HOW EJACULATING WORKS

When a man gets aroused, tubes in the penis known as the vas deferens squeeze out sperm from the testicles (testes) to the posterior part of the urethra. Fluids are also released from the seminal vesicles. The mixture of the sperm and fluid is subsequently sensed by the urethra, which, in turn, sends a stimulus to the spinal cord, at the height of sexual pleasure. The spinal cord subsequently sends signals to the penile muscles. The muscles there contract every few seconds. This contraction causes the semen to be forced out of the penis during the climax. In some cases, the scrotum becomes tightened during erection, and the foreskin is retracted automatically to reveal the glans. But in some men, the foreskin is retracted manually when the automatic retraction doesn't occur.

Men with erectile dysfunction are unable to have erections, and thus no ejaculation takes place during sex. Sometimes erections are spontaneous and not only as a result of sexual attraction, and some men with ED can achieve this type. Nocturnal Penile Tumescence (NPT) is the erection that occurs during sleep or when waking up from sleep typically in the morning. This kind of erection is mostly used to distinguish between the different types of erectile dysfunction. Be it the physiological or psychological type of erectile dysfunction.

SYMPTOMS OF ERECTILE DYSFUNCTION

Several factors come to play where ED is concerned. Early symptoms of the disease include but are not limited to:

• A reduced or lack of interest in sex

• Difficulty in getting an erection

• Severe challenges in maintaining the erection during sex or foreplay

There are some other sexual disorders which are related to erectile dysfunction; and just like ED, they can be a real nuisance during sex. They include:

• Delay in ejaculation

• Ejaculating Prematurely

• The inability to reach climax or orgasm even after ample stimulation (Anorgasmia)

CHAPTER TWO
PHYSIOLOGICAL CAUSES OF ERECTILE DYSFUNCTION

The study of erectile dysfunction in the medical field is known as andrology, which is a sub-field under urology (the study of the urinary tract and its diseases). Andrology is the male counterpart to gynecology as it deals with the male reproductive organs and its defects. But it isn't as detailed as gynecology, so they're still some uncharted territories within this area of study.

ED occurs when the parasympathetic nerves release an insufficient amount of Nitrous oxide (NO) to the penis. In most cases, it has been observed that, men over forty years of age experience one form of ED or the other.

There are two mechanisms involved in penile erection: the psychogenic erection, which is attained by emotional and erotic stimuli and works in line with the limbic system of the brain; and the reflex erection, which is as a result of the direct touching of the penis. This reflex erection uses the lower parts of the spinal cord and peripheral nerves.

For a complete and satisfactory erection to be achieved, the neural system must be intact and without damage. When the nervous system stimulates the penile shaft, Nitrous oxide is secreted, which then causes the smooth muscles of corpora cavernosa (penile tissue) to relax; and as a result of this relaxation, the penis becomes erect.

Additionally, the testes produce adequate levels of testosterone which is required for the healthy development of the erectile system.

Erectile dysfunction can be as a result psychological and physiological variables in the body, and both types can be treated.

PHYSIOLOGICAL CAUSES OF ERECTILE DYSFUNCTION

This type of ED can be as a result of an underlying condition or accident. Some common causative factors for this kind of ED include:

Diabetes, obesity, high blood pressure, atherosclerosis, multiple sclerosis, renal diseases, vascular diseases and chronic alcoholism. And neurological problems such as trauma from prostatectomy surgery, hypogonadism (hormonal insufficiencies), and side effects from some drugs, are also common causative factors. Sometimes drugs used for the treatment of lithium and paroxetine might also lead to erectile dysfunction.

The best way to know if ED is physiological or psychological is if during masturbation an erection can't still be achieved, or even during nocturnal tumescence a man fails to have or to sustain an erection. If it is psychological, an erection can be obtained during masturbation or when waking up from sleep, but not when with a partner. In cases where ED occurs physiologically, an underlying cardiovascular disease might be the root of the problem.

1. ENDOCRINE DISEASES

The endocrine system of the body produces different hormones that regulate various body functions like metabolism, reproduction, and sexual functions amongst others.

A major type of endocrine disease that causes erectile dysfunction is diabetes. It disrupts the body's ability to make use of the hormone called insulin. Chronic diabetes results in nerve damage in most cases. The nerve damage affects the sensations received by the penis and often impairs the flow of blood and hormone levels in the man.

2. NERVE AND NEUROLOGICAL DISORDERS

Different types of neurological disorders can result in the risk of increased levels of erectile dysfunction in men. The neurons act as messengers of the Central Nervous System and relay messages to and from it. Neurological disorders affect the ability of the CNS to communicate with the reproductive system and send signals to the penile muscles to achieve an erection.

Some common neurological disorders that often result in erectile dysfunction include:

▪ Parkinson's disease

▪ Alzheimer's disease

▪ Stroke

▪ Multiple sclerosis

▪ Brain and spinal tumors

In some cases, individuals who undergo prostate gland surgery may suffer from nerve damages as a result of complications during the operation. This damage might lead to erectile dysfunction if left untreated.

Also, the nerves in the buttocks and genitals might become weakened as a result of intense cycling in long distance riders. The repeated pressure on the nerves in this region could cause temporary impotence in the male rider.

Also, injury to the pelvis, spinal cord or penis, could require surgery, and when complications arise as a result of this, ED could develop.

3. MEDICATIONS

Some drugs can affect the flow of blood to the penis, and therefore it might cause erectile dysfunction in the patient if a large dosage is administered frequently. Some known drugs that cause erectile dysfunction include; diuretics such as furosemide and spironolactone, CNS stimulants like amphetamines or cocaine, CNS depressants such as Valium, Xanax, and Codeine, alpha-adrenergic blockers and beta-blockers, as well as cancer chemotherapy medications like Cimetidine.

4. ALCOHOLISM AND SMOKING

Alcoholism as a cause of erectile dysfunction is usually a short defect. Most times the individual recovers from the effects of the alcohol once it has passed. Since alcohol is a depressant, consuming a large quantity of it can dampen sexual desire and make it tough to reach climax or even get an erection. Too much alcohol affects both the penis and the brain. The blood flow to the organ is reduced significantly.

In cases where alcohol intake is chronically heavy, the erectile dysfunction becomes long-term. The combination of alcohol and smoking increases the risk of erectile dysfunction drastically. Studies based on research carried out show that, men who smoke ten or more cigarettes a day, have greater chances of developing ED; this is because smoking promotes the narrowing of the arteries.

Regardless of the underlying cause of ED; a doctor or specialist should be consulted immediately after detection. This is because ED can be treated quickly in its early stages.

CHAPTER THREE
PSYCHOLOGICAL CAUSES OF ERECTILE DYSFUNCTION

The psychological causes of ED are related to the state of mind of the man. It could be as a result of depression, anxiety, stress, relationship problems or other factors. This type is less frequent than the physical one and can be easily remedied. Researchers have noticed a strong response to the placebo treatment of this form of erectile dysfunction. This is because, most times, the mind can be manipulated into believing certain things.

In cases where the man is just shy and suffering from 'sexual anxiety,' the best way he can be put at ease is if the partner does not panic or get angry. It's usually advised that the partner should take charge of the situation and try to encourage the man. Take his mind off the situation by ramping up the foreplay or watching something provocative together. Most times, when he becomes at ease with himself and his partner, he will begin to get aroused, and his erection will follow.

HOW TO KNOW WHEN ED IS PSYCHOLOGICAL

If the man can get an erection during masturbation but cannot get it up during sex with a partner, then it's most likely psychological (stress related).

In most cases, the psychological factors are responsible for about 10-20% of all ED cases. It is often found to be a secondary reaction to an underlying physiological cause.

CAUSES OF PSYCHOLOGICAL ERECTILE DYSFUNCTION

▪ Anxiety

In some situations where the man has experienced problems in the past with getting it up, he tends to worry that it would happen again. This mentality often leads to performance anxiety or fear of sexual failure, and eventually, this could result in ED.

▪ Stress

If the man is stressed it could affect his performance in the bedroom. The stress could be finance-related, job-related or even because of the relationship. Several factors can cause stress related ED, and the best way to get rid of it is through relaxation.

▪ Guilt and Depression

In some cases, the man might feel guilty over something; it could be that he was unfaithful to his partner and cannot get over his guilt. Or maybe he just feels like he does not satisfy her enough. As a result of the split state of his mind, the brain cannot send the appropriate signals to his penis. Depression which is a common cause of ED can affect a person both psychologically and physically. Most times it can even cause a healthy man who's never had problems getting it up before to develop ED. And drugs used to treat depression can also result in erectile dysfunction.

▪ Low Self-esteem

The feeling of inadequacy in men as a result of several factors can also lead to ED.

▪ Indifference

Most times this can arise as a result of age and the subsequent disinterest in sex, due to different medications or relationship problems.

▪ Post-traumatic stress disorder (PTSD)

This type is mostly found in veterans and people that have gone through traumatic ordeals. PTSD impairs the sexual functions like desire, arousal, satisfaction, orgasm, etc. This type of ED can be cured when the disorder has been treated properly.

CHAPTER FOUR
SEXUAL PERFORMANCE ANXIETY

When sex becomes challenging and lacks its appeal for you or your partner, then it is most likely that anxiety is the problem. Sex is meant to be a fun and pleasurable experience, but it becomes a chore when you have performance anxiety. You're always questioning yourself, wondering if you're good enough for your partner or if she's enjoying herself. Your mind becomes too preoccupied with negative thoughts to enjoy having sex.

Constantly worrying about appearances and or sexual prowess with your partner can make sex nerve-wracking and stressful. Most times, it can even put you off from having sex entirely. Since sex is more than just a physical response, and arousal is mostly tied to emotions, when your mind is too occupied or stressed out to concentrate, your body will not get excited either.

Many things can cause performance anxiety. Some major ones include:

❖ Problems in the relationship

❖ Body image concerns

❖ Worrying that your penis wouldn't measure up

❖ The fear of ejaculating prematurely

❖ Not being man enough for your partner

Experiencing just one of the above factors is bad enough, but when the man has most of those fears at the same time, it is bound to result in ED. These anxieties cause the body to launch into the 'flight or fight' mode in response to the situation. Neurotransmitters such as epinephrine and norepinephrine are released by the body to confront the threat or run away from it. These anxieties usually result in the man being either aggressive or withdrawing from his partner, thus making intimacy between them difficult.

The state of your mind plays a significant role in arousal. Even if your partner is a very attractive person and you keep worrying about whether you'll be enough for her, the chances are that you'll end up not being able to perform or do so poorly. The stress hormones play different roles in men, one of which is the ability to constrict blood vessels. This constriction results in less blood flowing into the penis which makes it difficult to attain an erection. While sexual performance anxiety is mostly associated with men, it can also be found in women too, even though it is rare. Anxiety can prevent lubrication in women, thus eliminating the desire to have sex with a partner.

Sexual performance anxiety is usually in a perpetual cycle. You become so anxious about having sex that you end up under-performing. And then this fear leads to more stress every time you're about to have sex.

HOW TO OVERCOME SEXUAL PERFORMANCE ANXIETY

If you develop performance anxiety, the best thing to do is to talk to your doctor, or someone you're comfortable with for advice. The first thing your doctor will do is to run some tests on you to determine if there's an underlying medical condition involved. During the examination, the doctor might ask you about your sexual history and how long you've been experiencing this anxiety. Most times he'll want to know what kinds of thoughts invade your mind during or before sex.

Once it has been established that there's no medical related problem, then your doctor might suggest trying out a few of the following approaches;

• Seeing a therapist

Book an appointment with a certified sex therapist that's capable of handling your situation. You can learn to be comfortable with yourself through therapy, and also identify your issues. Once your problems have been addressed, they can then be eliminated or reduced. Men with premature ejaculation problems can be taught different techniques to control the situation. An example of methods used could involve humming or picturing something else to sustain the erection and delay ejaculation. Some therapists might even suggest counting to a hundred.

• Opening up to your partner

Confiding in your partner about your situation can help ease some of your anxieties. Coming up with a solution together can help the two of you to grow closer as a couple, thus improving your intimacy and sex life.

• Look for other means of distraction

Find new ways to distract yourself from your problem; like playing a sexy movie or music while having sex. Look for that film that turns you on or takes your mind off your problems. When you don't think about your issues for a little while, you'll find yourself growing excited eventually. Try not to beat yourself up if it doesn't work immediately, just give it time.

• Exercise more

Working out regularly not only helps to improve your health and state of mind but also improves your stamina during sex. Not only would you be physically fit, but you'll also feel better about how you look.

• Finding other ways to get intimate

There are some other ways to get intimate without having sex. You could take a warm bath with your partner or even give each other sensual massages. In other not to feel the pressure of performing sexually, you could always find more ways to pleasure each other. Most times oral sex gives the same amount of fun as coitus itself.

CHAPTER FIVE
LIVING WITH ERECTILE DYSFUNCTION

A study carried out by researchers showed that up to 30million men in America are affected by erectile dysfunction and that it increases with age. The disease affects about 12 percent of males below sixty, 22 percent of men in their sixties, and 30 percent of men aged seventy and above.

Even though the risk of ED increases with age, it is not inevitable for every male. The healthier you are, the better your chances of avoiding ED. Lifestyle choices are contributing factors of the disease and most times they can be prevented.

Diagnosis of Erectile Dysfunction

For your doctor to be able to ascertain the cause of your ED, a series of tests would have to be carried out. Some of the tests include:

• Physical Examination

This test is usually the first one performed, and it involves the doctor analyzing the penis and testicles to ensure they are in perfect working condition and the nerves are still intact. After that, he'll inspect your body for hair loss or abnormally large breasts, both of which are symptoms of hormonal imbalance. Your blood pressure would be taken, and your pulse rate noted.

• Urinalysis and Blood Tests

The outcome of your physical examination and your medical history would determine if the doctor needs to run blood tests or urine analysis on you. The tests would look for problems such as cardiac and renal (kidney) diseases, diabetes and problems with the hormones such as low testosterone levels. A different test would check your thyroid function.

• Nocturnal Penile Tumescence (NPT) Test

Also known as the Overnight erection test, it is used to find out if you can get an erection in your sleep. Usually, during REM sleep, men can have about three to five erections at night. NPT test is carried out by attaching a portable battery-powered device to the thigh while you sleep. The device detects the quality of your erections while you sleep and then records the data. In the morning your doctor analyzes the results and makes his observations known to you. A simpler version of this test makes use of a unique plastic ring, which will be placed around your penis. If you get an erection while sleeping; the ring breaks. NPT test rules out physiological factors as the cause of ED. It indicates to your doctor that your ED is as a result of a psychological factor.

• **Intracavernosal Test**

This test is also known as the injection test. Your doctor would inject a substance into your penis to induce an erection, but if you don't get one, there might be an obstruction to the blood flow in the penis. This procedure might indicate an underlying cardiovascular problem.

• **Doppler Ultrasound**

This method is used together with injection test and is also used to check blood flow to the penis. For the test, your doctor waves a wand-like device over your penis. This invention makes use of sound waves to create a video image of your blood vessels. Your doctor then uses this video to observe your penile blood flow.

• Examining your Mental Health

If after the other medical tests have been carried out and it looks like your ED is psychological, your doctor would have to ask you a series of questions regarding your mental state to find out the cause. These questions help him check for stress, anxiety or depression, which are leading causes of psychological erectile dysfunction. The doctor might also talk to your spouse or partner about your situation; to help him know more about your relationship and what's causing your problem.

HOPING AND COPING WITH ED

Erectile dysfunction can make a man to lose confidence in himself completely, get frustrated easily and sometimes even lash out at his partner as stated in the first chapter. While some men shy away from talking with their partners about their issue, it has been proven that talking it out always help to relieve the tension. Once your partner knows about the situation, it helps her understand what you're going through at the moment. You're not the only one affected by your condition; your partner is also affected even though it's indirect. The first step required in dealing with the disease involves being honest with yourself, your partner and then eventually your doctor. Once communication has been established, the next phase which includes diagnosis and treatment will be easy and less stressful because you have your partner's support.

It is also essential that you be very patient and cooperative while undergoing the treatment, and also keep in mind that the procedure you chose might not work immediately or might even have side-effects. So in this scenario, exercising patience is the best solution. Put your faith in your doctor and together, the two of you will work something out.

There are also support groups for men with ED to share their experiences and learn from one another.

Also, consider attending couple's counseling with your partner. It is essential that you don't shut out your partner during this period.

If it is your partner that has ED, you should try the following strategies;

➢ First of all, you should learn as much as you can about the disease, to better prepare you for the processes involved in handling it.

➢ Always show your partner affection and care, but don't smother him with it. Since he might be feeling touchy about his condition, you should always know when to take a step backward and give him space to breathe. Assure him that you'll have his back no matter what.

➢ Avoid keeping your feelings bottled up inside. Talk to your partner and tell him about your fears and concerns. Sharing things with him goes a long way in keeping the relationship alive and healthy. Also be positive minded and don't dwell on the bad stuff. Your positive attitude might help him feel less depressed or sad about himself.

➢ Adjust your sex life so that it would accommodate his new condition. Invent new ways to pleasure each other so as to reduce the pressure of him performing.

➢ Don't let him wallow in self-pity. Be his buddy and offer to go with him to his appointments even if he wants to go alone. Also, remind him always to update his doctor on any progress or new development.

➢ And finally, just have fun. Don't put much pressure on your partner or yourself. You could go on a vacation, sign up for a couple's massage or even yoga class, have a good time and just enjoy life as it is.

HOW TO RECOGNIZE DEPRESSION IN ED PATIENTS

The depression that usually comes with erectile dysfunction is treatable in most cases. Some key attributes of depression include: Feeling hopeless, persistent sadness and a pessimistic outlook towards life.

Depression symptoms include low self-esteem, fatigue, loss of interests in formerly enjoyable activities like sex, apathy, changes in appetite, thoughts of suicide and abuse of drugs and alcohol.

Since depression affects the way an individual feels about himself and life in general, treatments are usually required to help remedy the situation. The best-known treatments for depression are antidepressants and talk therapy. However, some antidepressants can worsen erectile dysfunction. So, the best way of preventing this is to alert your doctor of your condition so that he could prescribe safer drugs for you.

CHAPTER SIX
ELIMINATE SEXUAL DISTRESS FOREVER

As soon as you are diagnosed with ED, your doctor would have to determine the right form of treatment for you based on the nature of your condition; this is because the wrong type of therapy could worsen your state and make the disease harder to treat. Depending on the severity of the ED, your doctor might recommend various treatment options for you and your partner to choose. Your partner is included in the decision process because she also plays a role in your swift recovery.

Forms of treatment plans include:

Oral Treatments

Medications administered orally have a high success rate in the treatment of ED. The most popular type usually prescribed by doctors includes:

▪ Sildenafil (Viagra)

▪ Tadalafil (Cialis)

▪ Avanafil (Stendra)

▪ Vardenafil (Levitra, Staxyn)

Levitra starts working after thirty minutes and has a longer-lasting effect than Viagra. It lasts about five hours. Staxyn contains almost the same ingredients as Levitra, and it dissolves in the mouth, immediately acting after fifteen minutes. Viagra becomes active after thirty minutes and lasts for four hours. Cialis has a higher time frame than the rest; up to thirty-six hours in some situations.

The four medications listed above help in enhancing the effects of nitric oxide. Nitric oxide relaxes the penile muscles, which then causes the increase in blood flow and eventually the erection of the penis. These medications do not automatically induce an erection, but they help in the amplification of the signals that lead to the erection process.

Some of the medications might produce side effects in some men, which is why the doctor has to find the right type with the appropriate dosage for you. Some drugs might also be dangerous if taken alongside nitrate drugs, or if you have any cardiac diseases or low blood pressure.

The drugs should be stored in their original container and, in a cool and dry environment, away from heat and moisture. They should be kept out of the reach of small children and should be disposed of when not needed or if it's expired.

Injection Treatments and Suppositories

A fine needle is used to inject the drug Alprostadil into the side or base of the penis. Sometimes other drugs are mixed to produce a greater effect. This type of mixture is known as a Bimix or Trimix. This kind of medication provides an immediate effect immediately after it has been administered.

In the case of suppositories, the drug is placed inside the penis via the penile urethra, with the aid of a specially made applicator. This method has side effects like minor bleeding and pain in the urethra, the formation of fibrous tissue within the penis.

In some situations where a thyroid problem causes the ED, testosterone replacement therapy is recommended.

The Use of Penis Pumps

If it is observed that your medications aren't working as well as they should, then your doctor would recommend other means. One of such methods includes the use of the penis pump. It is also known as a vacuum erection device. The device is a hollow tube with a battery or hand powered pump. It is placed over the penis, and the pump is used to suck out the air inside the tube; creating a vacuum which draws blood from your body into the penis. Once an erection has been attained, a tension ring is slipped around the base of the penis to maintain the blood flow. This erection lasts long enough for you and your partner to have sex. The ring is to be removed after coitus. A side-effect of this method is the possibility of bruising to the penis and restriction of ejaculation as a result of the band on the penis.

Surgical Penile Implants

This method is usually used as a last resort because there could be complications involved during the process. The implants are placed on both sides of the penis. They could either consist of inflatable or bendable rods. The implants usually produce a high degree of satisfaction among men that have used them.

Exercising Regularly

It has been proven that vigorous exercise, especially aerobic ones, help improve erectile dysfunction. Men with cardiac conditions are advised not to overdo it. Exercising the body regularly helps in lowering the risks associated with ED. Your doctor should choose the right form of exercise suitable for your condition.

Counseling

As has been stated before in this book, counseling plays a significant role in the improvement of psychological factors behind ED.

Ayurvedic remedies

This type of medicine is a holistic and whole-body approach to health. It originally started in India, and it involves the use of herbal components to treat the disease. Some of its medication includes the use of the following;

• Indian Ginseng: it helps to regulate hormone levels and improves mental clarity by reducing stress levels.

• Asparagus Racemosus: this herb cures various types of diseases as well as improving blood circulation.

• Safed Musli: it helps in boosting sperm counts.

• Cassia cinnamon: a particular type of extract from the bark of an evergreen tree found in some regions in India. It improves sexual function.

Yoga is also a sure-fire way of reducing stress levels and helping in ED. It combines concentration, meditation, stretching, improving blood circulation and reducing the stress levels. Yoga has been shown to provide healthy levels of testosterone.

While these herbs have proven to be a success, it is also recommended that your doctor should give the green light before you go the herbal route, since little is known about the right dosage to administer.

Other Unconventional Methods

A new and controversial form of sex therapy has been discovered and is known as sex surrogacy. It involves pairing up patients with professionally trained sexual partners, who help them different disabilities. Some of which include; anxiety attacks, autism, physical disabilities, PTSD, schizophrenia, vaginal spasms and erectile dysfunctions. It helps with intimacy issues. This kind of therapy is a form of couple's therapy, for people who don't have partners. Once a surrogate is assigned to a patient, they meet in an open place and establish contact. After the initial contact has been established, the couple moves on to a green room where sessions of ninety minutes take place. Sessions may last for months or even a year. Sex surrogacy is more prevalent in Israeli than in other countries.

Conclusion

It's not going to be easy: it's certainly not. However, with the right treatment plan and a proper support system, you can still have a healthy and satisfying sex life. The condition can be tackled if you judiciously follow all the instructions given by your doctor and avoid harmful substances that could aggravate your condition. Following the actionable tips listed in this book will also help you a great. Since psychological erectile dysfunction occurs mostly because the mind is stressed out, therapy and support from loved ones always play key roles in its elimination. Never be ashamed to talk about your problem. Don't hold anything back.

It is important that you talk to your doctor before you attempt any of the medical options in the market. Some drugs and tools may not be suitable for you. The first step should always be diagnosing the problem, discovering the underlying cause and selecting a treatment plan.

Gynecomastia

Key Guide for Understanding Testosterone, Progesterone, Estrogen Hormones & Treatment for Male Boobs

Table of Contents

Introduction

Personal appearance can be a significant cause of anxiety in men and women alike. Conditions that impact appearance can be distressing and can lead to an altered sense of self, especially if this change in appearance leaves the individual looking or feeling different from others in their age group or social demographic. Gynecomastia, although common, is a frequent cause of male dissatisfaction with their appearance. Some men feel that the physical changes associated with gynecomastia cause them to look more feminine.

Gynecomastia is the name for the increased development of breast tissue in men. In spite of popular misconceptions, gynecomastia is actually common and even normal in men in certain age groups. By definition, gynecomastia is benign, although it can sometimes result from or be indicative of more serious conditions like cirrhosis of the liver or cancer. Gynecomastia can result from a number of different causes, including conditions of varying severity, so pinpointing the inciting trigger of gynecomastia in men is important.

Just as there are many causes of gynecomastia, there are also many treatments. Sometimes the treatment is as simple as removing the inciting factor. A thorough workup by the physician at the time the patient comes in will help him, or her determine what the inciting trigger is. Some men may choose to result to surgery if their gynecomastia is severe enough or particularly distressing, even in cases where the gynecomastia may resolve on its own. As the reader will see, many cases of gynecomastia (and most cases in adolescents) resolve without any need for treatment. In reality, the psychological effects of gynecomastia vary from one individual to the next, with some men being particularly bothered by it while other men or not.

As might be expected, gynecomastia is closely related to hormone levels in the bloodstream. This is why gynecomastia is more common in infants, teenagers, and adult men over the age of about 50 than it is in men of other ages. Physical changes in men can be closely tied to the levels of testosterone and estrogen-related hormones, and this is just as true of gynecomastia as it is of other physical states that men might experience. Gynecomastia is sometimes referred to as "man boobs," reflecting the perception that men have that the proliferation of tissue in their breast region causes them to look more feminine.

Men referring to gynecomastia as "man boobs" represents the reality that men commonly compare themselves to other men, leading men to feel shame at an appearance that instantly distinguishes them as being different from other men, even if it is in a superficial way. This comparison happens in many settings where men congregate with other men, whether it be in the locker room, at the gym, or other settings. The truth is that "man boobs" are much more common than many men realize, with about half of all adolescents and many men above the age of 50 experiencing it.

It could be argued that calling the condition "man boobs" marginalizes the men who go through it, causing them to feel more isolated from their peers. There has been an increasing emphasis on male appearance in the last 20 years, which may cause gynecomastia to be more distressing as it may represent for many a significant deviation from the norm, at least the norms that men see in television in media. Because gynecomastia causes male breast tissue to take on a softer, more feminine appearance, this condition becomes significantly more perturbing as it challenges the self-belief of these men that they are actually men. Of course, the reality is that images that men see in the media and associate with being manly or masculine often represent a reality that does not represent most men or is unattainable by most men. This will be discussed further in the fifth and sixth chapters of this book. This discussion delineates the much of the gynecomastia story is in the eye of the beholder.

But there is much more to the gynecomastia story than meets the eye. Doctors classify gynecomastia many different ways (based on severity and cause), and gynecomastia development is reflective of the rather complex interplay that sex hormones have on the male body. The purpose of this book is to educate men and women interested in gynecomastia on what the condition is, what causes it, and the effects that gynecomastia can have on the men that suffer from it. The different ways in which gynecomastia is classified will be reviewed in order to define what it is and what causes it. By providing an in-depth review of gynecomastia, the reader is placed in a position to adequately understand all aspects of the subject.

Understanding gynecomastia begins with clearly defining it, including learning the scales that doctors use to classify it and determine treatment. The severity of gynecomastia can vary so wildly that many men may not even realize that they have it, especially boys in the adolescent age group. This is an age where boys are often comparing themselves to their peers, and a boy with significant breast development can easily feel that he is very different from the other boys. It is normal for teenage boys to produce small amounts of estrogenic substances, but it is an excess production of these substances that leads to gynecomastia, which can be very significant if the hormone levels are greatly deviated from normal ranges for that age. This will all be explored thoroughly in the first chapter.

Classifying gynecomastia involves going on defining it, especially as many different types of doctors deal with gynecomastia, and many of these have come up with their own ways of measuring severity. Gynecomastia is often the preserve of the family doctor or internist, but radiologists, surgeons, and others are often involved. In the second chapter, the medical classification of gynecomastia will be discussed along with how the primary doctor makes the diagnosis and proceeds with his or her medical workup.

Truly understanding gynecomastia requires a basic understanding of sex hormones in the male body. A discussion of what the normal male hormones are and how those hormone levels vary by age is key to really getting a feel for why gynecomastia happens and how it can be treated. Sometimes gynecomastia development is as simple as a medication slightly shifting the balance between testosterone and other hormones, a shift that is enough to tip the edge in favor of the proliferation of glandular tissue around the male breast.

Another important issue to explore regarding male sex hormones is how altering the normal balance of your sex hormones, through the addition of testosterone, for example, can lead to conditions like gynecomastia. This is the case for men who take anabolic steroids, hoping to increase size, strength, or both. The effects of exogenous testosterone use can be very dramatic, but the long-term consequences can be serious. Excess testosterone is readily converted to estrogenic substances by the body, making anabolic steroid use a major factor leading men to obtain gynecomastia removal surgery. Indeed, unlike some other causes of gynecomastia, breast tissue proliferation that results from anabolic steroid use is generally not reversible. Gynecomastia is relatively common in this community and the term "man boobs" may be more familiar to some anabolic steroid users than the more technical gynecomastia. The important and interesting role that anabolic steroid use has on the gynecomastia story will be explored in the third chapter.

Gynecomastia can have natural or physiologic causes, or it can result from conditions or factors that males do not normally experience, which is called nonphysiologic. The distinction between the two is important for medical professionals to make as part of their determination of how the gynecomastia that surfaces should be treated, or if it should be treated at all. It is important that a physician does not attribute gynecomastia to a natural process when it may reflect a more serious medical condition. The medical community is well aware of this and they have come up with a process of properly working up gynecomastia. There are also notable ethnic differences in proliferation of male breast tissue, especially in the adolescent age group. Both of these topics will be explored.

The effects of gynecomastia can be long-lasting. Although some men choose not to have their gynecomastia removed (even if it is irreversible), they can still experience depression, shyness, and social phobia as a result of their unique physical appearance. The psychological effects of gynecomastia can be very dramatic, which is part of the reason why some doctors recommend removal in some patients.

Gynecomastia (and the underlying hormonal changes that it represents) can also affect other areas of a man's health, such as his libido. Sex drive is an important part of being a man, and concerns about libido represent one of the main reasons why some men go to the doctor about their gynecomastia. Gynecomastia may be a condition that is closely associated with a feminized appearance, but many men are just as concerned about their testosterone levels and the implications that this has on other aspects of their life as they are on the physical manifestations of gynecomastia itself. The psychological and sexual effects of gynecomastia will be discussed in the fifth and sixth chapters.

Abnormal male breast tissue can be surgically removed, or it can be treated in other ways. Whether or not a man decides to get treatment can be impacted by a number of different factors, including suitability for surgery, whether or not the gynecomastia is likely to go away on its own, what the cause of the gynecomastia is, and the man's willingness to undergo surgery. Sometimes the choice of whether or not to treat gynecomastia is not the man's own. Fortunately for many men, surgery is not the only option. The various treatment options for gynecomastia will be discussed in chapter seven.

By understanding gynecomastia, the reader is equipped to be supportive of men that they know that may be experiencing gynecomastia and are concerned about it. The reader himself may be experiencing the condition and curious to learn more. In this book, they will learn not only the ins and outs of gynecomastia, but the long and detailed story having to do with sex hormones in the male body. There is a lot to gynecomastia, but a careful study of the subject does equip the reader to filter through all the noise on the internet and in the media. With this knowledge, the ruler can truly gain a sense of what this gynecomastia subject is all about.

Chapter 1: What Is Gynecomastia?

Testosterone is a subject that many men obsess about. This is just as true of younger men interested in increasing their testosterone as it is for older men faced with issues of declining testosterone. It seems that testosterone has (in the minds of many men) a life of its own. It is something that can be increased or decreased by various factors. Some men seem to think that testosterone gets up and walks away at a certain age. Although many men have misconceptions about testosterone, the idea that gynecomastia and other physical changes that men may experience has something to do with testosterone is not a misconception.

Indeed, testosterone (and estrogenic compounds as well) is an essential piece in the gynecomastia puzzle. Gynecomastia can result from an abnormal balance of sex hormones in males. With the increased emphasis on male appearance that is obvious to most men, what was once a little-discussed subject has become a frequent topic of discussion on television, on the internet, and on other media where information is disseminated.

Modern men are bombarded with images of archetypal men. These men are muscular, have low body fat, and are shown to have the favor and appreciation of the women around them. These men with their bulging pectorals, biceps, and six-pack abs are presented as if they are the norm for men. Indeed, the idea that these almost superhuman images represent a small subset of men is a topic in and of itself, but it is an important one to at least touch on when dealing with the subject of gynecomastia.

Gynecomastia has likely been around for as long as men have been around so why the sudden interest in this condition now? Standards of masculinity have changed across the ages and they have long varied in the various cultures of the world, but there does seem to be a convergence in the image of masculinity that both men and women see in the world today, regardless of their background. In short, men all the world over are being faced with images and ideas of masculinity that have changed. Whether you live in the United States, United Kingdom, Russia, India, or South Africa, you are likely to be faced with an image of masculinity that places more emphasis on the appearance of men than perhaps was the case in the past.

Men are expected not only to deal with the demands of a changing world, including changing roles for men in society, but they are also expected to look a certain way, a look that may be unachievable for many men. There is no question that this increased emphasis is not only responsible for the increased use of anabolic steroids and other performance-enhancing drugs by men, it is also responsible for men perhaps caring about their gynecomastia more than ever before. Adolescent men with minor gynecomastia that is likely to go away on its own in a year or two are going to their doctors wondering if they can have their hyper-proliferated breast tissue removed. This is also true of men in the 50 and 60-year-old demographic, who perhaps were less concerned about their chest appearance in the past.

Gynecomastia, therefore, represents not only a medical condition that can be both physiologic and non-physiologic in men; it reflects a changing consciousness in men that their appearance is important. Many men feel the depression or anxiety that comes from their gynecomastia, but they do not perhaps understand that these feelings they feel (and even how they perceive themselves) come from societal forces that are not under their control.

That tackles the issue of why gynecomastia is important, but what is gynecomastia. Gynecomastia is the term for the proliferation of breast tissue in males. Men generally

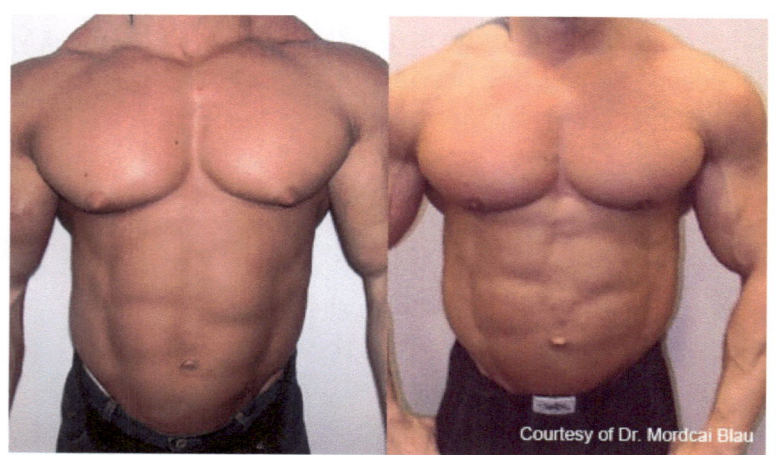
Courtesy of Dr. Mordcai Blau

have minimal glandular and adipose tissue in the breast region, particularly around the nipple. This is especially true if a comparison is made between an anatomically typical male and a woman. By definition, gynecomastia occurs in males as healthy, non-obese men do not typically have lasting, significant glandular or adipose tissue in the breast. The increased appearance of tissue in the region of the male breast is called gynecomastia, and it is not uncommon for it to crop up in men in certain age groups. In fact, about one-half of all adolescent men, primarily between 13 and 17, will experience some breast tissue development that ultimately disappears.

Breast tissue that develops in adolescent males typically goes away within six months to two years after onset. This is the case in what is known as physiologic gynecomastia. That is, gynecomastia that is considered to be a normal part of development as opposed to gynecomastia that is caused by a medication or medical condition. Although most adolescent physiologic gynecomastia goes away, it has become increasingly common for young men in this age group to express an interest in surgery to treat their gynecomastia

The first important concept to note in the gynecomastia discussion is the distinction between physiologic and nonphysiologic gynecomastia. There are several ways in which gynecomastia can be delineated or described, but this particular breakdown is an easy and approachable way to understand gynecomastia from the standpoint of its causes. It is also an important way for the medical provider to approach whether or not the gynecomastia that he or she is seeing is part of a normal life change or if it is aberrant.

- Physiologic gynecomastia: Age-related proliferation of breast tissue. It is not caused by a medical condition or by medication and it has a trimodal age breakdown.
- Nonphysiologic gynecomastia: Gynecomastia that results from a medical condition, medication, or illicit substance. Nonphysiologic gynecomastia has a number of causes and does not result from age-related hormonal changes.

Physiologic gynecomastia has a trimodal breakdown in terms of the age of the men impacted, which means that it normally surfaces in men in three age ranges: newborns less than four weeks of age, adolescent males between 13 and 17, and men above the age of 50. Physiologic gynecomastia is called this because it can be considered a relatively normal part of male development, as opposed to nonphysiologic gynecomastia that is due to causes the fall outside the realm of natural development.

Physiologic gynecomastia is believed to represent about 25% of all cases of gynecomastia, leaving the other causes with a large share of the responsibility for the prevalence. This should not come as a surprise when one considers the large numbers of medical conditions or medications that can result in gynecomastia. As non-physiologic gynecomastia essentially represents all causes of gynecomastia that do not occur as the result of natural changes in hormone levels related to age, it should come as no surprise that most causes of gynecomastia fall under this umbrella.

The major causes of gynecomastia are listed below:

- Chronic renal insufficiency
- Cirrhosis of the liver
- Genetic condition
- Hyperthyroidism
- Idiopathic cause (unknown)
- Infection
- Medication
- Primary hypergonadism
- Secondary hypergonadism
- Tumors

Among the potential causes of gynecomastia, some are more common than others. Medications as a cause of gynecomastia represent 25% of cases as does gynecomastia that is of unknown cause (idiopathic). Gynecomastia that develops in a male that is not in one of the age groups associated with physiologic gynecomastia and who has no other known cause would be classified as idiopathic by the medical provider (although a cause for the gynecomastia may later be discovered).

Primary and secondary hypergonadism are important causes for gynecomastia, representing together about 10% of cases. Hypogonadism refers to decreased size and function of the testes, and the distinction between primary and secondary hypogonadism has to do with whether the cause of the hypogonadism comes from within the testes or has to do with a cause outside of it. Even within the category of secondary hypogonadism, there are a number of distinct causes that together comprise about 8% of all cases of gynecomastia.

Some of the causes of primary hypogonadism include injury or abnormal anatomy like testicular trauma or testicular torsion. Some genetic causes fall under this umbrella as well, such as 5-alpha reductase deficiency and Klinefelter syndrome, although there are also genetic causes of gynecomastia that do not involve hypogonadism. Infection, hemochromatosis, and viral orchitis can also be causes of the proliferation of breast tissue in males via hypogonadism.

The role that organ dysfunction has on gynecomastia should be noted. Cirrhosis of the liver and chronic renal insufficiency are both major causes of gynecomastia, with cirrhosis alone representing an estimated 8% of all cases of gynecomastia. It may come as a surprise that chronic organ conditions can cause a hormonal condition of this magnitude, but the liver and kidney both play important roles in hormonal balances in men both as sites of production of hormones and as sites for hormone removal.

Tumors are a serious cause of gynecomastia, and it is important for a medical professional to rule these out when making their determination as to the cause of the gynecomastia. The normal diagnosis of gynecomastia involves more than just a physical exam with close examination of the breast tissue, it involves obtaining hormone levels in the blood and it may also involve imaging. Hormone levels, in particular, can be very important as the presence of particular hormones, or hormone levels that are extremely high may indicate the presence of a serious tumor that will require further investigation.

Although it may be easy to fall into the trap of attributing gynecomastia in an adolescent male to physiologic gynecomastia, the presence of a large amount of breast tissue, as well as other medical complaints that the adolescent male may have, may make it necessary for a doctor to investigate further. Because some of the causes of gynecomastia are very serious and may be life-threatening, further testing is often indicated even if the first inclination of the doctor is to attribute the gynecomastia to natural changes in hormone levels (physiologic gynecomastia).

The number of medications that cause gynecomastia is quite large. The list includes a number of medications that are commonly used, like phenytoin, haloperidol, minoxidil, diltiazem, finasteride, digoxin, and diazepam. Indeed, creating an exhaustive list is difficult because of the large number of medications that may be involved. Indeed, any medication that can cause an increase in testosterone or estrogen can theoretically cause gynecomastia, although the list of medications includes drugs that operate by a wide variety of different means.

The medication causes of gynecomastia can be broken down by method of action; that is, by how specifically they cause the proliferation of breast tissue. As has been mentioned in the book already, any medication that alters the concentration of testosterone or has estrogenic action can cause gynecomastia. The major categories of medication-induced gynecomastia are listed below:

- Estrogenic action (increases estrogenic hormones)
- Androgenic action (increases androgenic hormones like testosterone)
- Increases the concentration of sex-hormone binding globulin
- Increases the breakdown of androgens
- Causes production of prolactin
- Unknown cause

Much to the dismay of doctors, many of the most common medication causes of gynecomastia work by action that is as yet unknown. This include some common medications like ACE inhibitors (angiotensin-converting enzyme inhibitors, amiodarone, and amphetamines. The reality is that most medications that are prescribed by doctors have side effects, and any medication that has even a covert action on hormone levels could potentially cause gynecomastia. The list of medications that cause this condition is likely to increase as more medications reach the market and as more patients report their symptoms to their medical providers.

Recreational drugs can also cause gynecomastia. This includes drugs that operate as opiods and opiates, like heroin and methadone, as well as marijuana and amphetamines. When one takes into account how different medications interact with each other, the possibility for increased hormonal dysfunction leading to gynecomastia and other conditions is almost endless. Even alcohol can be a cause of gynecomastia, both secondarily as a cause of liver cirrhosis, or as a primary factor that induces the breakdown of androgenic compounds like testosterone.

There is much more to the story of the causes of gynecomastia, including the complex pathway by which hormones interact with each other. Further exploration of the subject is best left until the role of hormones in males (normally) is explored. Certain foods like soy have even been blamed for the development of gynecomastia, although the concentration that is linked to breast tissue proliferation in men is relatively high. Within the domain of gynecomastia and its causes is the question of which causes result in irreversible gynecomastia – that is, gynecomastia that does not go away when the trigger is removed. Gynecomastia that is caused by a medication is often irreversible.

Chapter 2: Types of Gynecomastia and Diagnosis

Gynecomastia is also categorized by the histological changes that it can cause in men; that is, the changes at the cellular and tissue level that will be apparent in cytological examination and on diagnostic imaging. These types are often referred to as phases as they represent increasing degrees of severity of tissue changes. Normal male breast tissue contains ducts below the areola. It is similar to the breast tissue of girls before puberty. The phases or types of gynecomastia are based on changes in this basic normal appearance. The phases are:

- Nodular (or florid) phase
- Dendritic phase
- Diffuse phase

By categorizing gynecomastia in this fashion, doctors are able to correlate the severity of the gynecomastia with the imaging that they obtain (if the physician is concerned enough that they decided to obtain imaging). The physician is then able to have an understanding of the proliferation of the breast tissue relative to how the chest usually appears. Much of this topic is the domain of radiologists, although this categorization does help the primary care doctor to better understand how far along the patient is in terms of their condition.

As stated above, male breast tissue normally contains ductal and epithelial cells below the areola, just like pre-pubertal girls. Nodular phase gynecomastia is associated with the proliferation of these ducts as well as of epithelial cells. The ducts have been stimulated to increase in number by the imbalance of estrogenic and androgenic hormones. In short, testosterone has decreased relative to the estrogenic (female) hormones. Nodular phase gynecomastia is generally reversible.

The second phase of gynecomastia that is important is dendritic phase. Dendritic phase gynecomastia is associated with a change in the appearance of the ducts rather than a mere increase in number. Ducts in this phase will appear dilated and there may also be some fibrosis (formation of hard tissue). These changes will be visible on diagnostic imaging or on cytological examination, although imaging should be enough to make the distinction.

Diffuse phase gynecomastia is more serious than the other types. It may contain features of both dendritic and nodular phase gynecomastia. The male breast in diffuse phase gynecomastia often closely resembles a female breast. There will be dense breast tissue and there may even be lobule formation. Lobule formation is highly abnormal in men and raises concerns for more serious pathology. Making the distinction between these types of gynecomastia can be important for the primary care doctor (or radiologist) to determine where the male is in terms of the severity of their condition and whether or not the condition is likely to be reversible. This topic will be discussed further later on in the book.

The Gynecomastia Scale

There is yet a third way of classifying gynecomastia. This comes from the American Society of Plastic Surgeons. This is based on the appearance of the gynecomastia from the standpoint of the surgeon who will be tasked with removing it. This classification takes into account the involvement of the proliferated breast tissue with the surrounding areas, and particularly the extent to which the areola is involved. More severe gynecomastia, from the standpoint of this scale, involves significant enlargement of the breast with excess or redundant skin. This classification is defined as follows.

- Grade I: enlargement of the breast with localized tissue underneath or around the areola
- Grade II: moderate enlargement of the breast with tissue boundaries that are not easily distinguishable from the chest
- Grade III: moderate enlargement of the breast outside the borders of the areolar region, and with excess or redundant skin
- Grade IV: moderate enlargement of the breast with excess or redundant skin and significant female appearance to the breast

This classification of gynecomastia is based on a modification of earlier scales and represents how the American Society of Plastic Surgeons currently classifies gynecomastia based on severity. This classification is associated only with gynecomastia, as conditions that do not represent benign proliferation of male breast tissue are excluded.

Diagnosis of Gynecomastia

Gynecomastia is by definition benign, which means that a serious condition like a primary cancer of the breast is technically not gynecomastia. The doctor, therefore, has to rule out more serious concerns in order to make the diagnosis of gynecomastia. A critical part of the diagnosis of gynecomastia is the history and physical examination obtained by the doctor or medical provider. Physicians who are reviewing the case of a male coming in for gynecomastia need to take into account the major categories of causes, making sure that they obtain information about each in order to rule them in or rule them out. For example, because gynecomastia can be caused by medication or illicit drug use, a thorough and honest history of medications used will be very important in ruling out medication as a cause.

It is important that physiologic causes of gynecomastia are expected to resolve either when the adolescent leaves the teenage years or after two years of onset, so gynecomastia that has persisted longer than this duration is a major cause for further exploration by the doctor. The point being that a doctor should not attribute gynecomastia to physiologic cause in a male who has had unresolved gynecomastia past the age of 18 or for more than two years.

There are other findings that the doctor may make on his history of physical examination that may cause him to proceed to imaging or laboratory workup right away. During the physical examination, the doctor needs to eye the breast tissue to determine if it is unilateral or bilateral. It is also important for the doctor to palpate the breast tissue to determine the nature of the tissue. Gynecomastia is usually present in the area of the areola. This area will be palpated to determine if the tissue in the region is glandular or fatty. Fatty tissue under the areola may not be gynecomastia, while glandular tissue is more likely to be gynecomastia, though it can also be a cyst, infection or inflammation (mastitis), or a tumor.

Based on his or her physical examination findings, the doctor will determine if the gynecomastia can be attributed to a natural or physiological cause related to age, or if there is another cause that is potentially more serious. Nonphysiologic gynecomastia will typically require a work up with diagnostic imaging and/or lab testing. Again, the history will help guide the doctor here. If the patient reports a medication that commonly causes gynecomastia, like an antipsychotic or anti-depressant medication, the doctor may perhaps only obtain lab work. Diagnostic imaging is especially useful to rule out a tumor or any other mass that does not feel like typical adipose of glandular tissue.

It is possible that the doctor may aspirate the area to obtain some cells for examination, although current guidelines suggest that this should only be done if the doctor is concerned about a tumor. The purpose of viewing the cells under a microscope would be to determine if the cells are tumorous, as tumors are medical emergencies that need to be investigated urgently. Another portion of the physical examination is also a testicular examination. This is to determine that the abnormal breast findings are not also associated with abnormal testicular findings. On physical examination, the doctor may not know the presence of hypogonadism or a testicular mass, both of which would provide valuable information to the doctor as to the cause of the gynecomastia. Based on these findings, the doctor would make a decision as to how to proceed. Again, a testicular finding would lead the doctor to obtain imaging of that area just as he would if he found a mass suggestive of a tumor in the breast.

Once the doctor makes the determination that the patient has gynecomastia that is not physiologic or due to a common chronic disease like cirrhosis of the liver, the doctor then has to further investigate with lab work. Lab work will test for the presence of specific hormones. If a particular hormone is particularly high or particularly low, the doctor will be able to determine what the likely cause of the gynecomastia is. For example, high levels of human chorionic gonadotropin and prolactin are suggestive of tumor, while low levels of testosterone are generally indicative of hypogonadism (whether primary or secondary)

Diagnostic imaging is a common way for a physician to investigate what he suspects to be the cause of gynecomastia. The imaging the doctor orders will depend on the area of the body that he is concerned about. A tumor in the breast will generally lead to a mammogram and ultrasound of the breast. Concern for a testicular mass will result in an ultrasound of the testes. A concern about a pituitary tumor will lead to a magnetic resonance imaging scan (MRI) of the pituitary to rule that out.

Conditions that Need to Be Distinguished from Gynecomastia

There are a number of conditions that a physician will need to distinguish from gynecomastia on physical examination and as a part of his workup. As has been mentioned, male breast tissue normally contains ducts below the areola but is not normally associated with excess fatty tissue, lobules, or significant fibrosis (hardening). If the doctor discovers these on his examination, he or she should start thinking about what else could be happening in the male breast that may not be gynecomastia.

Gynecomastia is benign by definition, which means that it is not a life-threatening condition. The reason why it is, therefore, important to make a distinction between gynecomastia and other conditions is that some of these conditions are in fact life-threatening so making the right diagnosis early can be critical. There are in fact a number of conditions that may be superficially similar to (or mistaken for) gynecomastia, but these would be easily distinguishable to a radiologist on diagnostic imaging. Some of these conditions include:

- Lipoma: fatty growth that is generally more fibrous in men than in women and commonly mistaken for gynecomastia
- Cyst: well-circumscribed fluid filled sac
- Myofibroblastoma: a type of growth that contains fibrous muscle tissue
- Angiolipoma: a type of growth that consists of adipose tissue mixed in with blood vessel development
- Inflammatory lymph node: a normal lymph node that has become inflamed. May be associated with more severe condition or prior history of cancer in the breast region
- Fat necrosis: a mass of fatty tissue without the typical histology of normal adipose cells
- Hematoma: a blood collection that may be associated with prior trauma to the chest
- Seroma: a fluid collection that may be associated with prior surgery to the area

- **Retropectoral abscess:** an infection below the pectoralis muscles that has formed an abscess
- **Male breast cancer:** (see below)

Male breast cancer is a serious concern that will have to be worked up by the doctor. The majority of masses found in the male breast are not breast cancer, especially in men in the trimodal age ranges associated with physiologic gynecomastia. This does not mean that the doctor can ignore this. Therefore he may resort to imaging in the form of a mammogram or ultrasound in men who have breast development that is atypical for physiologic gynecomastia. This includes men with firm breast tissue, other health complaints, or a family history of breast cancer.

Again, most proliferation in the male breast is not breast cancer. It is not the goal of this book to frighten the reader into worrying about cancer. This is merely a part of the normal workup by the doctor. The biggest concern that men generally have when it comes to gynecomastia is resolving the appearance of the area so that it can resemble the normal chest appearance in a man. Some men refer to gynecomastia as "man boobs," and this highlights the underlying concerns that men have that their chest makes them look or feel feminine.

The male chest is an important representation of male strength and power; at least it is in the minds of many men. In Classical times, it was normal for great leaders to be portrayed with monumental statues that often depicted them as having larger than life qualities, often in the form of a muscular appearance. One of the most typical aspects of that muscular appearance was a strong, powerful chest. The typical appearance of the male chest is one of the characteristics that readily distinguishes males from females. By emphasizing or exaggerating the chest in statues, the sculptor underlined the point that the person portrayed was a man with masculine or even hypermasculine qualities.

As modern society has become more visually-oriented, there has been an increase in emphasis on male appearance. Many men may have been exposed to images when they were growing up (in the form of cartoons, movies, comic books, and other visual media) that planted an idea in their minds of what a normal man looks like. It is important to note that these sorts of ideas are not specific to individual men, but are societal. As much as one may be inclined to attribute male dissatisfaction with their appearance to an internal psychological problem (like body dysmorphic disorder) it is certainly the case that societal expectations of men have changed. Men may be expected to pay more attention to their appearance now than they might have in the past. Some men may be more immune to these influences than others, a subject that will be discussed further later on in the book.

In addition to concerns about the appearance of their chest relative to other men, a man may have worries that the presence of gynecomastia may be indicative of an underlying problem with their testosterone levels. This worry about testosterone can be regarded as distinct from concerns about appearance as testosterone itself (and the testosterone level) may be associated in the minds of some men with virility and power (or lack thereof). This is a subject that will be discussed further later on in the book.

It is part of the diagnostic workup of men who do not have physiologic gynecomastia to have their hormone levels checked. Again, it is normal for men in the trimodal age ranges of physiologic gynecomastia to have a relative increase in estrogenic compounds relative to testosterone. This may be associated with a total decrease in testosterone or with an increase in both testosterone and in estrogenic compounds as is the case with adolescent males. The interplay that these hormones have with one another is complex. It is important to understand these hormones and to get a picture of why "man boobs" develop in the first place.

Chapter 3: The Role of Hormones in Men's Health

Men of the 21st century are paying closer to attention to their hormone levels, particularly testosterone, than ever before. As men have become increasingly more concerned with appearance, sex drive, and masculinity, they have also devoted more of their time and energy towards ways of increasing or otherwise manipulating their testosterone levels naturally. For some men, this means resorting to foods or drugs (like anabolic steroids) that may increase the level of androgenic hormones in the blood, while for other men it means taking advantage of their relatively high testosterone levels that they can.

Indeed, a fixation on testosterone has become so common in the United States in this decade that hundreds of thousands of men have gotten their testosterone levels measured for the purposes of being given exogenous testosterone by their doctors. Although testosterone is a controlled substance in the United States (as it is in most countries), it is medically indicated in men who are found to have low testosterone after a test that carefully measures testosterone at certain times of the day. Therefore, many men are able to receive testosterone safely without worrying about developing complications.

But testosterone prescription by a doctor is not the subject of this chapter or this book. This really is a chapter about testosterone itself, along with the other androgenic and estrogenic substances that comprise the normal balance of hormones in the male bloodstream. Most men reading this who are interested in learning more the role that hormones play in men are curious about the subject because they recognize that it is the key to understanding gynecomastia. Indeed, the subject of gynecomastia cannot really be understood unless one has some understanding of male hormones as all causes of gynecomastia (with the exception of conditions in the male breast masquerading as gynecomastia) are related in some way to levels of androgenic and estrogenic substances in the bloodstream.

Therefore, understanding both the causes and the treatment of gynecomastia requires some understanding of normal sex hormone function in men. This is a complex subject to discuss because it is not as simple as merely having gasoline in your car or not. Hormone levels not only fluctuate with age, but they even vary based on time of the day. This makes understanding the subject somewhat trying for the layperson, but also challenging for the physician when it comes to making the right diagnosis. With that said, it is possible to make statements about hormone balances in men that are true and which help to make the subject of gynecomastia more approachable for the average person.

Testosterone

The hormone most closely associated with masculinity and male characteristics is testosterone, although the picture surrounding this and other hormones is complicated. For example, testosterone is present in hormones in mothers during pregnancy, with both male and female fetuses being exposed to it. Women also have levels of testosterone present in their bloodstream during various periods in their lives, while men normally produce and are exposed to levels of estrogenic compounds like estradiol during some phases in their life. Although some studies have linked testosterone to aggression and competitiveness, it has been shown that estrogenic substances like estradiol also can cause aggression, and women are actually more sensitive to testosterone than men are.

Testosterone is a steroid that, like other steroids, is synthesized from cholesterol in several steps. Testosterone is able to accomplish its action by activation of androgen receptors through bindings. Testosterone is normally produced in the testes of men, although some testosterone is also produced at time (but to lesser extent) in the female ovaries. Males are also exposed to sex hormones that are produced in the mother or by the placenta during gestation and after birth.

It may come as a surprise to some, but testosterone is present to some extent in females as well as males, although levels of testosterone in males are almost 10 times greater than what they would be in females. Production of testosterone is even greater than that ratio suggests as testosterone is actively turned over in males, requiring more production. Normally, most testosterone is bound to plasma proteins with only about 2% of testosterone being unbound. Many factors can influence normal testosterone levels in otherwise healthy men including exercise, weight loss, vitamins and nutrients, certain foods, and sleep.

The role of testosterone in men and women is actually relatively complex. For example, it has been found that the subjective experience of love reduces testosterone levels in men, but increases testosterone levels in women. Although males generally have more total testosterone than women, the differences in amounts of free testosterone may be less dramatic as women typically have less bound testosterone than men, especially during pregnancy.

The reality is that normal sex development and sexual characteristics in men and women has as much to do with the relationship of various hormones to each other rather than the presence or absence of hormones. This is very true in the case of gynecomastia, in which the issue is often the elevation of certain estrogenic substances relative to testosterone than it is the absolute level of testosterone. Indeed, older men with gynecomastia tend to have an issue with lower overall testosterone while adolescent men with gynecomastia often have an elevation of testosterone and estrogenic compounds like estradiol.

The discussion of male hormone can be approached from the standpoint of an exploration of testosterone, a discussion of what hormones are normally present in men, and an exploration of how disturbances in the relative levels of these hormones can lead to conditions like gynecomastia. This issue of hormone disturbances will be addressed in particular in terms of the trimodal distribution in age that characterizes physiologic gynecomastia: namely neonates, teenagers, and men above 50.

During pregnancy, the effects of testosterone on the fetus vary depending on the stage of the pregnancy. Very early in the pregnancy, testosterone stimulates the formation of structures that will eventually form the characteristics of males, such as the scrotum, the phallus, and other structures, although the impact is thought to be less than that of another compound called dihydrotestosterone. Although these structures begin to form early on (including the seminal vesicles and prostate gland), true sex characteristics as a result of testosterone exposure do not appear until later. Testosterone exposure in the second trimester is thought to impact both male and female sex characteristics.

After birth, male infants have essentially pubertal levels of testosterone for a period of several months, although these levels eventually drop to hardly detectable ranges. They will rise again when the male enters puberty. This fall in testosterone at about six or seven months is not clear, although it may allow males to develop other biological characteristics as a result of a relative increase in other hormones relative to testosterone. In other words, testosterone may be taking a wee bit of a break and then reappearing leader to virilize males.

Science has yet to fully understand the complex interplay of hormones like testosterone during infancy. It is known that the so-called masculinization of the brain is due to both testosterone and estrogen. Although male brains are larger and have more neural connections during adulthood, it is believed that the transformation of testosterone into estrogen and the entry of estrogen into the male brain is associated with male brain development. This process is different in females as estrogen is typically bound to a protein called alpha-fetoprotein and prevented from entering the brain.

Therefore, masculinization appears to be due to female hormones as well as male hormones, with females frequently being exposed to male hormones, and female hormones occasionally being blocked in females at certain times. This is part of what makes the gynecomastia discussion so interesting: the issue of hormones is not a straightforward question of whether you have testosterone or not. Although the effects of testosterone are often mitigated by other hormones, like estradiol and other estrogenic compounds, the medical profession can summarize (and has) the general impact that testosterone is thought to have on males.

- Muscle growth
- Increased bone density
- Increased strength
- Linear growth of bone
- Bone maturation
- Maturation and of the penis and scrotum
- Facial hair growth
- Axillary hair growth
- Vocal deepening

The effects of testosterone can be divided into anabolic effects and androgenic effects. Anabolic effects are associated with muscle growth, increased bone density, and strength. These are the effects that many men who take anabolic steroids illicitly are interested in obtaining. Testosterone can also cause the so-called androgenic effects, which include sexual maturation, voice deepening, hair on the face, chest, and under the arms, and other sexual secondary sex characteristics. It is these characteristics that physically distinguish males from females. These characteristics are associated with the changes that males undergo after puberty.

The effects of testosterone during puberty include those listed above along with others that are associated with enduring masculine characteristics, as well as the changes that male adolescents experience during this time. This includes increase in libido, growth in genital size, bone growth in the face (especially the chin, brow, jaw, and nose), closure of growth plates and cessation of growth, broadening of shoulders, enlargement of the Adam's apple, expansion of the rib cage, and growth of the sebaceous glands, which leads to acne.

Some other common and well-known effects of testosterone include growth in pubic hair, growth of hair in other regions (including on the chest, on the legs, and under the arms), loss of fat in the face, and loss of hair on the scalp. Some of the effects of testosterone occur indirectly via metabolites of estradiol, for example, the closure of the growth plates. Because of the role that estrogenic compounds play here, the period of growth tends to last longer in men than in women, leading to a gradual cessation in growth rather than a sudden stop.

The impact of testosterone (even leaving aside the idea that testosterone's role is mitigated by other hormones) is therefore complex. Although testosterone has been associated in some studies with aggression and antisocial behavior, it has also been found that testosterone is associated with fairness and justice, as men with higher testosterone are thought to treat others more fairly than those with lower testosterone. But the social effects of testosterone are somewhat outside the scope of this book.

The last subject to discuss regarding testosterone is the idea of changes in testosterone levels that occur. It has been mentioned already that testosterone levels can fluctuate during different age ranges, but testosterone also fluctuates during the day. Testosterone is generally highest first thing in the morning, so levels of testosterone measured for diagnostic purposes are generally measured then. This is not only to obtain an accurate testosterone measurement, but also to compare this measurement to established normal levels that have been determined through studies.

An important subject for the man or woman learning about gynecomastia to learn is that of the role testosterone plays in gynecomastia, both physiologic and nonphysiologic.

The Role of Hormones in Physiologic Gynecomastia

Physiologic gynecomastia that occurs as the result of normal hormonal fluctuations of hormones like testosterone with age is arguably the single most common cause of gynecomastia. The good thing for men who fall into this category is that gynecomastia that is due to natural hormonal changes is benign and either resolves or does not have consequences of lasting import. A common group that experiences this type of gynecomastia is adolescents and their gynecomastia generally resolve within a couple of years of onset or by the age of 18. But what causes this gynecomastia in the first place?

Like any question having to do with the role of hormones in gynecomastia, the answer is complex. It would be simple if it were merely a case of low testosterone, but that is far from the truth. Indeed, in neonates (or newborns), gynecomastia is due to the presence of estrogenic compounds from the placenta and from the mother in the bloodstream. It may surprise some to learn this, but the mother's own hormones are present not only in the fetus but in the newborn and have important and lasting effects. Although gynecomastia in infants sometimes is disturbing to parents, this gynecomastia generally goes away within a few weeks.

As discussed previously, gynecomastia in adolescents is very common. This type of gynecomastia is associated with Tanner stage three or four, or about 13 or 14 years old. This type of gynecomastia is associated with a relative increase in estradiol and a relative decrease in free testosterone production. Male tissues during this period become increasingly sensitive to estrogenic compounds. Complicating physiologic gynecomastia in adolescents is the reality that males in this age range can also experience nonphysiologic gynecomastia due to foods, medications, illicit drugs, or medical conditions. A common discovery during this age is actually genetic conditions that were hitherto unnoticed.

The final group that is subject to the effects of physiologic gynecomastia is men over the age of 50. This can also be confused with nonphysiologic gynecomastia, but when it is physiologic, it is due to a drop in free testosterone. This is normal for men in this age range, as this period is often referred to as andropause, but a host of other factors can also lead to a reduction in testosterone. Studies have suggested that fatherhood and child rearing also lead to a drop in testosterone in men, although these benign causes of testosterone falls are not due to underlying medical problems and therefore can contribute to rather than confuse physiologic gynecomastia.

As mentioned in the first chapter, medications are among the most common causes of gynecomastia with some estimating that as much as 25% of gynecomastia may be due to medications, tying it for first place with physiologic gynecomastia. Most (if not all) causes of gynecomastia resulting from medications have to do with the effects that these medications have on hormonal balances in men. The hormonal situation in men is already relatively sensitive to changes under normal circumstances so it is not difficult to imagine that any change caused by a medication can have dramatic results.

As touched on briefly previously, medications can affect the normal hormonal balance in men in various ways. Hormones can interfere with the ability of androgenic compounds like testosterone, or they can have estrogenic properties. Hormones can lead to the breakdown of androgenic compounds like testosterone (thereby reducing the free concentration of testosterone), or they can reduce free testosterone by increasing the concentration of proteins that bind to testosterone. They can also lead to an increased concentration of prolactin, a hormone that causes lactation and can also lead to ductal proliferation around the areola. Finally, medications can act by unknown mechanisms to lead to gynecomastia. It is important to note that drugs like marijuana and heroin can also cause gynecomastia, and these are often listed under medication-related causes of gynecomastia rather than being listed as a separate category.

Progesterone
Progesterone is a hormone that is normally present in both men and women. In men, progesterone is produced in the testes, although levels are lower in men than in women. Progesterone in men, as with women, serves as an important intermediate steroid in the production of other steroid hormones.

Chapter 4: The Causes of Gynecomastia

The causes of gynecomastia are numerous. Leaving aside the case of physiologic gynecomastia, gynecomastia can be caused by medications, illicit drugs, medical conditions, or even the consumption of certain foods. This means that the medical professionals tasked with diagnosing gynecomastia often have their work cut out for them as they must tease out whether the gynecomastia is due to a natural hormonal change (that may resolve itself) or due to something more serious.

Some of the main causes of gynecomastia are listed below:

- Chronic renal insufficiency
- Cirrhosis of the liver
- Genetic condition
- Idiopathic (unknown)
- Hyperthyroidism
- Impaired absorption (cystic fibrosis, ulcerative colitis)
- Infection
- Malnutrition
- Medication
- Primary hypergonadism
- Secondary hypergonadism
- Tumors

Arguably the three most significant causes of gynecomastia are physiologic, medication, and unknown, which together make up about 75% of gynecomastia. An entire book can be written about the medications that cause gynecomastia, as they are many and varied. As many men and women in the United States are on a number of different medications, gynecomastia in men can be the result of a single medication or of several, rendering the pharmacological picture quite complex.

Some of the well-known medications that can result in gynecomastia are:

- Venlafaxine
- Theophylline
- Risperidone
- Reserpine
- Rosuvastatin
- Nifedipine
- Minoxidil
- Methyldopa
- Fluoxetine
- Fenofibrate

- Diltiazem
- Atorvastatin
- ACE Inhibitors
- Antiretroviral drugs
- Amlodopine
- Haloperidol
- Phenytoin
- Diogixin
- Spironolactone
- Omeprazole
- Methotrexate
- Ketoconazole
- Flutamide
- Cimetidine
- Amphetamines
- Amiodarone

Atypical Causes of Gynecomastia

There are a number of less common causes of gynecomastia that can make pinpointing the cause difficult. Malnutrition can be a cause of gynecomastia as can conditions that result in malabsorption. This can be due to both the reduced production of hormones as well as the suppression of hormone production. Typically, resuming a normal diet that includes all the necessary vitamins and nutrients is able to resolve gynecomastia that arises as a result of malnutrition. This may not happen immediately as the liver plays a role in this recovery. The liver is responsible for breaking down estrogens and may take up to two years to recover from malnutrition.

There are several conditions that can cause malabsorption. Malabsorption is the general term for the poor absorption of nutrients, vitamins, and minerals in the gut. As the reader can imagine, any condition that causes the appearance of the gut to be abnormal can lead to malabsorption, along with a number of other conditions. Of the conditions that can cause gynecomastia as a result of malabsorption, cystic fibrosis and ulcerative colitis are among the more prominent.

Another cause of gynecomastia is obesity, although obesity is more closely associated with what is known as pseudogynecomastia. Pseudogynecomastia is male chest tissue that appears feminine due to the presence of fat in the area rather than the ductal (glandular) tissue that is associated with actual gynecomastia. Obesity can actually cause true gynecomastia because the presence of excess fat in men is associated with hormones that lead to an increase in estrogenic compounds.

As a roundup of the atypical causes of gynecomastia, it can be mentioned that infection of the testes can result in gynecomastia, as can exposure to harmful metals like lead. Infection or trauma to the testes can lead to gynecomastia by impacting the ability of the testes to produce normal levels of testosterone. Human immunodeficiency virus can cause gynecomastia either directly or indirectly because of antiretroviral drugs. Finally, nearly a quarter of all men have gynecomastia of which the cause is not known.

Ethnic Differences in Gynecomastia

There can be ethnic differences in the development of gynecomastia as well. This is due to ethnic differences in circulating testosterone concentration as well as androgenic compounds. African-American adolescents may develop gynecomastia because of elevated testosterone levels compared to other adolescents. This elevated testosterone may be aromatized to estrogenic compounds, leading to a relative reduction in free testosterone as compared to these estrogenic compounds.

This picture is also complicated by the obesity epidemic in some countries. Gynecomastia may be diagnosed more frequently in countries or communities where obesity is more common. This may be attributed to the misdiagnosis of pseudogynecomastia as gynecomastia, or because of the effects that fat has on hormonal balances. Thus, obesity clouds the picture of ethnic differences in gynecomastia as it can make it difficult to pinpoint whether adolescent gynecomastia is more prevalent in some groups as compared to others.

Hypogonadism

Primary and secondary hypogonadism are major causes of gynecomastia. In fact, these are categories rather than specific causes as they encompass a number of conditions that can result in reduced size or function of the testes. These conditions may overlap with other causes of gynecomastia, especially as some of these conditions or genetic. Also, malignancy itself can cause hypogonadism, therefore creating in these males two causes of gynecomastia rather than just one.

Hypogonadism refers to the reduced function of the testes, which can lead to a reduced production of sex hormones like testosterone. Sometimes hypogonadism in males is referred to as hypoandrogenism, although the term hypogonadism appears to be more common. The reduction of androgen production in males may be responsible for much of the physical aspects that we associate with hypogonadism (and gynecomastia), although there are a number of other hormones that can be impacted. Some of the hormones that may also be reduced include inhibin, DHEA, and activin.

Although hypogonadism is important to discuss as a cause of gynecomastia, this particular finding may be the least of the worries of men who fall into this category. Hypogonadism often leads to reduced sperm production (or no sperm production), which can make it difficult or impossible for men with hypogonadism to produce offspring. Men with hypogonadism may experience impaired libido, often with no interest in sex at all.

Making the diagnosis of hypogonadism in males involves testing testosterone and luteinizing hormone. The levels of these hormones are standardized based on age in order to make appropriate assumptions about what the levels mean. Primary hypogonadism (hypogonadism due to a defect in the testes itself) can be due to conditions like Klinefelter Syndrome, a genetic condition in which the individual has an extra X chromosome. Secondary hypogonadism can be due to a number of causes external to the testes, like hemochromatosis, or defects in the pituitary.

Chapter 5: The Psychological Effects of Gynecomastia

Why all the fuss about gynecomastia anyway?

Gynecomastia has been the subject of increased attention in part because men are becoming more concerned with their appearance and are more likely today to go to their doctor with their concerns than they were in the past. Although gynecomastia can be caused by medications and medical conditions that might make gynecomastia slightly more common than it may have been one hundred or two hundred years ago, men in the past were less likely to obtain surgery based solely on the appearance of their chest rather than an underlying medical condition.

The "fuss" about gynecomastia, therefore, has as much to do with the prevalence of the condition as it has to do with male perception of their own gynecomastia. As men have begun to be subject to a lot of the body concerns that women have, they have begun to place a greater emphasis on changing the appearance of their body to match the images that they see in print media, television, movies, and other forms of media.

The Various Causes of Psychological Symptoms in Gynecomastia

Gynecomastia can lead to more than just a feminized appearance to the chest. It can also lead to depression, social phobia, and shyness as a result of men feeling that they are less of a man because of their appearance. Although the case has been made that masculinity has been damaging to men by causing themselves to perceive their role in ways that are (arguably) dysfunctional to themselves and to others, the reality is that human beings operate based on social groupings and it is normal for people to know their role in the group by comparing themselves to their peers. Men, therefore, develop a sense of what it means to be a man by comparing themselves to other men. This is true of women, as well, and it is also true of whatever other social groupings that someone may choose to analyze.

The psychological effects of gynecomastia are complicated as gynecomastia can result in a type of situational depression, in which a man is depressed or down because of the development of gynecomastia, but it can also be a depression that has another cause. Depression in men with gynecomastia can be due to hormone imbalances related to the gynecomastia. Depression can also be related to whatever the underlying cause of the gynecomastia is, be it a medication, medical condition, other triggers.

For example, some antidepressant and antipsychotic medications can lead to gynecomastia. A doctor may see a patient who comes in complaining of a feminine appearance to his chest. After obtaining a history, the doctor realizes that the man is 52 years old and has a history of alcohol abuse and is also taking an antidepressant medication. This man's gynecomastia may be related to his age, his alcohol use, the medication that he is taking, or all three. Also, if this man is depressed, is it because he is usually depressed because his hormone levels are abnormal due to his underlying liver condition because his medication dose is too low, or because of another yet unknown reason? This illustrates how complex gynecomastia can be, not to mention how layered the situation can be when other complaints like psychological matters are taken into consideration.

The psychological issue can be really broken down into three main areas relevant to gynecomastia. The first is the body dysmorphic disorder that men may be experiencing because of an increased emphasis on male appearance. Body dysmorphic disorder is defined as a distorted image of oneself that causes dysfunction. Individuals with eating disorders often have a body dysmorphic picture associated with their illness. Body dysmorphic disorder has become more common in men because of images that men are seeing and that they are interpreting as normal when the images actually represent atypical representations of maleness and masculinity.

The depression or other psychological effects of gynecomastia can also be due to hormonal changes associated with the gynecomastia itself. Low testosterone can lead mean to feel depressed or emotional. This is not an issue caused directly by the gynecomastia, but it is one that is related to the hormones associated with the gynecomastia.

Finally, psychological symptoms with gynecomastia may be related to the underlying cause, leaving aside the hormones. For example, a medication or medical condition can be causing the depression, things like hypothyroidism. The psychological picture, therefore, can be broken down into the following three things:

Psychological symptoms due to situational depression.

Psychological changes due to hormonal changes.

Psychological changes due to non-hormonal cause of gynecomastia.

Chapter 6: Anabolic Steroids and the Sexual Effects of Man Boobs

Summary of the Sexual Effects of Gynecomastia

Related to the psychological discussion of man boobs is that of the sexual effects. Because gynecomastia is closely tied to levels of androgenic and estrogenic compounds in men, sexual effects of gynecomastia are often tied to hormones rather than a condition resulting directly from the gynecomastia itself. Indeed, gynecomastia is itself a benign condition. Gynecomastia does not itself lead to other symptoms, although other conditions associated with it can.

Gynecomastia can be tied to a decrease in sex drive in men. This can be as a result of the psychological aspects of the gynecomastia, or because the underlying cause of gynecomastia is also causing a libido issue. Medications that cause gynecomastia can also lead to reduced libido. This makes determining the cause of the gynecomastia an important step in resolving the physical aspects of the gynecomastia as well as the psychological and sexual effects. Remove the cause of the gynecomastia and resolve the appearance of the male chest and there is a great chance that both the sexual and psychological effects will disappear.

The term "man boobs" gives an idea of how some men regard gynecomastia, whether that gynecomastia effects them personally or it impacts other men. These "man boobs" are often due to anabolic steroids, although about 25% of gynecomastia is due to medications of which anabolic steroids are a major component. In reality, minor gynecomastia is often ignored or undetected, leaving the major cases of gynecomastia to be referred to as man boobs. This leads us to a discussion of the role anabolic steroids play both as a cause of gynecomastia, and as a cause of other symptoms.

Anabolic Steroids

Anabolic steroids are a common cause of gynecomastia. These are compounds that may be prescribed by a doctor or which may be taken illicitly in order to enhance performance or to change appearance. Although many readers may associate anabolic steroid use with professional sports or bodybuilding, many Americans today who take anabolic steroids have actually been prescribed these compounds by their physician.

There are a number of reasons why anabolic steroids may be prescribed by a physician. As mentioned previously, testosterone the hormone normally has androgenic and anabolic effects. The anabolic effects of testosterone include an increase in muscle mass, bone density, and strength. It is not difficult to understand why athletes of both sexes might resort to performance-enhancing drugs like anabolic steroids. They can give the athlete a competitive advantage in terms of strength and size, and this may be enough to give them the proverbial leg up on their competition in professional sports meets. Of course, amateur athletes may also engage in the use of performance-enhancing drugs like anabolic steroids.

Perhaps the most famous anabolic steroid users are bodybuilders, although the use of anabolic steroids is probably more common in other groups than people realize. A male user of anabolic steroid obviously uses these compounds to develop the extreme muscle hypertrophy that is necessary to win the major competitions that characterize this sport. Anabolic steroids have been used to improve appearance since the early 19th century, although they really took off in the 1950s and 1960s. It is not easy to pinpoint exactly why anabolic steroids became popular during their period, though it was probably related to the increased images of "strong men" on television and the movies that spurred the change. There was a benefit to men to use anabolic steroids as it would have landed them in movie roles, on television, or magazine covers.

It was around this time that bodybuilding competitions began to become more common and popular. Some men were inspired to begin bodybuilding because of the images of Venice Beach bodybuilders that they may have been exposed to in the 50s and 60s. It is easy to understate the role that images like those on television and movies play in human cognition, but when it comes to gynecomastia and anabolic steroids, the connection is pretty obvious. These images were subliminally teaching men what it means to be a man, and a lot of that had to with what men looked like. This will be discussed in more detail later, but men entered fields like bodybuilding (or used anabolic steroids) because of perceptions they had about what it meant to be a man.

The subject of the relative good or ill of anabolic steroids used for the purpose of achieving a masculine image is a subject onto itself, one that will be addressed in this book. Suffice it to say, anabolic steroids used for bodybuilding or appearance, in general, are a major reason why anabolic steroids are taken by men, and a major cause of gynecomastia. Indeed, it can be argued that until recently most gynecomastia surgeries were performed on males using anabolic steroids, and this may still be the case in some locales.

There are other reasons why men may be given androgenic compounds. In addition to being given to men in the midst of physiologic gynecomastia, androgenic compounds may be given to transgender men undergoing masculinization. Androgenic compounds have also been given to women with breast cancer to counteract the effect of estrogenic compounds.

The role that androgenic compounds taken exogenously has to do with gynecomastia is similar to the role that testosterone and other androgens play in the condition. Although there may be an increase in total testosterone, problems like the aromatization of testosterone into estrogen or a reduction in free testosterone may be associated with this state of androgen excess (not unlike what males experience in puberty). This is why men exposed to exogenous androgens get acne and virilized facial features just as adolescent boys might.

Anabolic steroids can actually lead to reduced libido in men, reduced sperm count, and disorders in sexual functioning. Although this may seem counterintuitive, prolonged exposure to elevated levels of testosterone in the blood often leads to hypogonadism, which results in abnormal sexual functioning in men. When one takes into account that excess testosterone can be converted into estrogen, is not difficult to see why anabolic steroid use can lead to a host of problems in men, including both gynecomastia and sexual dysfunction.

Chapter 7: Treatment of Gynecomastia

The first step to treating gynecomastia is determining the cause. Many men jump to the conclusion that the only treatment for gynecomastia is to remove the abnormal tissue, but many cases of gynecomastia are reversible and do not require surgery. Physiologic gynecomastia in adolescents does not require surgery as it is resolved naturally in the majority of cases. But this is not just true of adolescent gynecomastia. Gynecomastia that is due to a trigger, like a medication or medical condition may also resolve on its own, although it may not depending on the severity of the medication. Gynecomastia that is due to obesity or diet may also be reversible.

Examples of causes of gynecomastia that is unlikely to resolve on its own are gynecomastia that result from anabolic steroid use and gynecomastia that is severe (diffuse gynecomastia, or Type IV gynecomastia, depending on the scale you are using). Gynecomastia that resembles a typical female breast (that is gynecomastia that is very severe) is unlikely to resolve without surgery.

Surgery involves removal of the abnormal tissue associated with the proliferated breast. Surgery may be difficult if there is a significant abnormality in the region, although cases like these are more likely to be considered for surgery. The surgeon will attempt to remove as much of the ductal or fat tissue as he can while preserving as much of the areola and the normal pectoral appearance as possible.

Surgery may be contraindicated in certain cases. These are also cases in which insurance companies are unlikely to cover surgical procedures. These cases include:

- Gynecomastia that is likely to resolve without surgery
- Gynecomastia that results from hormone use (or abuse), or supplement use
- Gynecomastia that results from the abuse of alcohol
- Pseudogynecomastia
- Grade I gynecomastia (minor gynecomastia from a surgical standpoint)

There are some non-surgical treatments for gynecomastia. These include:

- Removal of the medication trigger
- Tamoxifen (medication)
- Raloxifene (medication)
- Clomiphene (medication)
- Dihydrotestosterone

Studies are divided about the efficacy of medication in men with gynecomastia that is not associated with malignancy, and more research may have to be done to further support the use of these medications.

Frequently Asked Questions

1. What is gynecomastia?

   Gynecomastia is the name for the presence of increased breast tissue in men. This breast tissue is in the form of adipose tissue (fatty tissue) and glandular tissue primarily around the breast. Gynecomastia, therefore, is associated with an appearance of the male chest that more closely resembles a female breast than the typical mal chest. In fact, the name gynecomastia is derived from the Greek and indicates a female-like chest.

   Gynecomastia has been covered extensively in the medical literature because its causes are varied. The effects that it can have on the man with it can also be varied. Many men who have gynecomastia did develop it because of natural, physiologic causes but as a result of a medical condition or a medication. Many men go to their doctors with their concerns about the appearance of their chest although not all men end up getting surgery. The presence of gynecomastia is closely tied to levels of sex hormones in men.

2. What causes gynecomastia?

   Gynecomastia is divided into two categories which essentially represent the two major classes of causes for the physical change. Physiologic gynecomastia is gynecomastia that results from age-related changes in male hormones rather than from an iatrogenic cause or a medical condition. Physiologic gynecomastia affects men in three age groups: newborn infants, teenagers, and men above the age of 50. These are all ages in which men are experiencing hormonal changes that do not reflect the normal state of male hormones (particularly testosterone) in the blood.

   Nonphysiologic gynecomastia is the name given to gynecomastia that results from a medical condition, a medication, or the abuse of an illicit substance. Many medications can cause gynecomastia, and this is a common cause for this condition in men between the ages of 18 and 50. This type of gynecomastia is not considered physiologic or "normal" in that men would only develop this type of gynecomastia if there is a problem causing their sex hormones to be abnormal. Both categories of gynecomastia are therefore related to levels of testosterone and estradiol in the blood.

3. Are there different types of gynecomastia?

   In addition to categorizing gynecomastia based on its causes, gynecomastia can also be divided into types based on its diffuseness and appearance. This allows doctors to assess the severity of gynecomastia relative to how the male chest normally appears. Gynecomastia can be divided into three phases or types. These types are nodular (or florid), dendritic, and diffuse. Male breast tissue normally contains ducts below the areola and is basically similar to that of girls before puberty. The male breast does not normally contain lobules.

   The nodular phase or type of gynecomastia is associated with proliferation of subareolar ducts and epithelial tissue. This means that the ducts have been stimulated to expand by an imbalance of androgenic and estrogenic hormones. The proliferation of ducts is in the nodular phase is associated with an increased number of ducts and is generally reversible. Dendritic gynecomastia is associated with dilation of ducts and fibrosis. This type of gynecomastia appears differently on cytological examination.

   Diffuse phase gynecomastia is the most severe type or phase. It has features of both nodular and dendritic phase gynecomastia. The changes are severe enough that the male breast will resemble the female breast in terms of density. There may be lobule formation (which is associated with men with serious complications like cancer) and this is highly abnormal in males. The different phases of gynecomastia are generally distinguishable on mammogram or ultrasound.

4. What hormones are responsible for gynecomastia?

   Much of male and female appearance is due to the presence of sex hormones in the blood. Indeed, normal male appearance is very closely tied to the level of testosterone and the presence of other hormones. In both men and women, these hormones engage in a complicated dance that results in what are called secondary sex characteristics, or the phenotypical appearance that generally marks a person as appearing male or female.

   Leaving aside the question of normal male appearance versus normal female appearance, the hormones that specifically play a role in gynecomastia are testosterone and estradiol, although other hormones like progesterone and prolactin can be important as well. Although many men and women may think that gynecomastia results from low testosterone, in fact, gynecomastia sometimes results from testosterone levels that are abnormally high which results in some of the excess testosterone being converted into estrogen.

5. Can anabolic steroids cause gynecomastia?

Related to the subject of the influence of testosterone on gynecomastia development is the role of anabolic steroids. Men take anabolic steroids in order to encourage strength or muscle development. Many different compounds are considered anabolic steroids, but they basically have in common that they are generally precursors of testosterone. That means that these compounds will be converted into testosterone in the body. Some men (and women) interested in size and strength choose to take testosterone itself rather than a precursor. Testosterone can also be prescribed to men who have been found by their doctor to have low testosterone.

The concern with testosterone is that excess testosterone is converted into estrogen in the human body. This is true of adolescent males as well as of men who take anabolic steroids or testosterone enanthonate (a formulation of testosterone). Males frequently have high levels of testosterone in their adolescent years (and into their 20s) and this testosterone is converted into estradiol, which stimulates the development of male breast tissue. This conversion also occurs in men who utilize anabolic steroids for performance, although other drugs can be added to prevent the development of gynecomastia in males taking performance-enhancing drugs.

6. Is surgery the only way to treat gynecomastia?

It is important to approach the treatment of gynecomastia from the standpoint of what has caused it in the first place. Physiologic gynecomastia, often seen in adolescent males, may not require treatment at all because if typically resolves within six months or two years of development. The severity of adolescent physiologic gynecomastia may vary widely, with some boys not realizing that they technically have gynecomastia. Physiologic gynecomastia can be treated if it disturbs the man or boy although generally is not required as it is benign.

Nonphysiologic gynecomastia is its own can of worms as it results from a specific cause rather than hormonal changes due to age. This type of gynecomastia may resolve or lessen in severity if the cause, such as a specific medication, is removed. Unfortunately, many causes of nonphysiologic gynecomastia cause permanent proliferation of abnormal glandular tissue at the site of the breast, so it is not uncommon for surgery to be resorted to. There are other treatments for gynecomastia, but when treatment is warranted surgery is generally considered the most effective way to treat.

7. If I get my gynecomastia removed is there a possibility that it will return?

Nonphysiologic gynecomastia may return even if the abnormal adipose and glandular tissue is removed. The goal of the surgery is general to remove all of the abnormal areas with the goal that the gynecomastia will not return, but if the man affected is exposed to the cause of the initial gynecomastia a second time it is possible that the gynecomastia will return.

An example of this would be a man who is exposed to exogenous sources of testosterone in the form of anabolic steroids. A man who has his abnormal breast tissue removed may develop gynecomastia a second time if he is exposed to anabolic steroids again. The goal of the procedure is to remove the glandular tissue and adipose tissue that has proliferated, but there is a possibility that not all of the tissue was removed and the site may develop a feminine appearance a second time around because of excess testosterone.

8. Can gynecomastia result in lactation?

A phenomenon that is sometimes seen in men that use anabolic steroids is gynecomastia with the development of functional breast tissue. The chest region may still have the appearance of hypertrophic pectoral muscles, but the glandular tissue is actually equivalent to female glandular tissue, which means that it responds to cues that trigger lactation. This means that males with gynecomastia can experience lactation if the production of milk is stimulated by the presence of another hormone, prolactin.

Prolactin is the hormone that normally stimulates milk production in breastfeeding mothers. Just as with typically male hormones, prolactin and other hormones have a complex relationship with each other with hormone levels rising and falling based on cyclical changes associated with uterine tissue and signals from the brain. Normally, prolactin levels fall when a mother stops breastfeeding which results in a cessation of milk production. In men, however, the prolactin levels are not tied to natural cues. The presence of lactation and high prolactin levels in a male will be detected by a doctor. The doctor or medical professional would then have to determine if this finding is associated with a medication or illicit substance (like an anabolic steroid) or if it is due to a more serious condition like a tumor.

9. Do I have to get my breast tissue removed if I have gynecomastia?

Recall that gynecomastia can be either physiologic or non-physiologic. Physiologic gynecomastia in a newborn or adolescent generally goes away after a period of time while gynecomastia in a male over 50 may not. Non-physiologic gynecomastia may or may not go away on its own depending on the cause. The first determination that the doctor needs to make is what the cause of the gynecomastia is and whether or not it is likely to resolve without surgery.

If there is a chance that the gynecomastia will resolve on its own without surgery, the doctor may recommend against surgical treatment. It is possible that a male may opt to have surgery anyway and many men with both physiologic and non-physiologic gynecomastia opt for surgery. Because gynecomastia is considered benign, even men with relatively severe gynecomastia have the option of surgery. The indication for male breast tissue removal would generally be if the tissue is not benign or if the doctor is unsure if it is benign or not.

10. Do men normally develop breast tissue?

The proliferation of glandular and adipose tissue is not typical for males, although men may experience the development of some breast tissue at certain times of their lives. This is the trimodal distribution of physiologic gynecomastia: newborn babies, teenagers, and men over 50. Some men never develop any form of visible breast tissue, although approximately 50% of male adolescents will develop some degree of gynecomastia. In many adolescents, this "breast tissue" is very minor and results in little or no discomfort or psychological symptoms in the male.

11. Can excess testosterone lead to the development of gynecomastia? Can gynecomastia affect my sex drive?

Excess testosterone that is converted into estradiol is a major cause of gynecomastia, especially in adolescents. This is also a major cause of gynecomastia in many men with nonphysiologic gynecomastia. A medication, medical condition, or illicit drug may lead to greater than normal testosterone levels that can result in excess estradiol as well. Although testosterone excess is a major cause of gynecomastia, it is not the only cause as certain medical conditions or drugs can also lead more or less directly to gynecomastia without the involvement of testosterone.

Men of all ages may report a decreased libido along with their gynecomastia. This is actually due to a number of factors. The levels of particular hormones in the blood may cause reduced libido, especially low testosterone and high estradiol. Reduced libido may also be related to the condition or medication associated with the gynecomastia, rather than to the hormones themselves. For example, certain medications that are given for psychiatric purposes may cause reduced libido in men as well as gynecomastia.

12. What is the gynecomastia scale?

The gynecomastia scale is a classification system that the American Society of Plastic Surgeons uses to characterize gynecomastia based on its severity. Yes, it is yet another way to classify this condition, although the approach is mainly from a surgeon's standpoint. The gynecomastia scale is divided into four grades based on how significantly enlarged the areolar breast tissue is, how much redundant skin is involved, and how close in appearance to a female breast the gynecomastia is.

Conclusion

The story of gynecomastia is a long one as it can appear with varying degrees of severity and for different reasons. Gynecomastia refers to the proliferation of breast tissue in men. This tissue is in the form of ductal or glandular tissue that leads to a feminized appearance to the male breast. Although it is not abnormal for ductal cells to be present in the areolar region on men, this tissue is generally minimal and does not result in a visibly feminine appearance to the male chest, which is normally categorized by relatively more muscle and less fat than women. Gynecomastia in men is categorized by a proliferation of this ductal tissue, which can be related to an increase in a number of these cells, the dilation of ductal cells, or both. Gynecomastia can vary greatly in severity.

Gynecomastia is a subject of concern for many men as they may be experiencing it personally or know someone who is. The single most common cause of gynecomastia is generally thought to be physiologic gynecomastia, which is due to normal fluctuation in hormone levels as a result of age. The men generally affected by physiologic gynecomastia fall in the age groupings of male newborns, teenagers between the ages of 13 and 17, and men above 50. But, as we have seen, this trimodal age breakdown is complicated by the many other causes of gynecomastia that can interact to cause men in these groups to have gynecomastia for another reason (or for their propensity for gynecomastia to be exaggerated for another reason).

As we have seen in the book, the discussion of gynecomastia is complicated by the many different causes of the condition, as well as the many ways that it can be classified. Gynecomastia can be classified as physiologic or nonphysiologic, or it can be described based on the appearance of the breast tissue on imaging (nodular, dendritic, or diffuse). Gynecomastia has also been described by surgeons based on the severity of the glandular growth and the superficial appearance of the area from a surgical standpoint. By this classification, gynecomastia can be divided into four types.

The causes of gynecomastia include medical conditions, tumors, drugs, genetic conditions, and substances in the environment. In spite of the many known causes of gynecomastia, one in four cases has been described as being idiopathic or of unknown cause. Because there are so many causes, a male may have gynecomastia for one or more reasons, making it even more difficult for the medical professional to pinpoint the cause.

Understanding gynecomastia requires an understanding of the normal balance of male hormones. In spite of what many have been led to believe, testosterone is present to some degree in both men and women. Also, estrogenic substances are also present in males to some extent. In fact, it is the balance of these hormones that leads to normal development in men and women from the fetal stages straight through adulthood. Indeed, it has been shown that estrogenic substances are responsible both for male brain development to some extent and for the normal process of growth during and after puberty.

Gynecomastia is an interesting subject not only because of its complexity but also because of the psychological effects that it has on men. Both men and women generally see themselves by comparison to their peers. This means that men make associations about what it means to be a man by looking at other men. Because gynecomastia is characterized by a feminized appearance to the chest, this condition may leave men feeling depressed or unmanly because they do not have what they regard as a typical male appearance. Although some may be inclined to say that it is dysfunctional for men to feel this way, it is the case that human beings have no innate sense of normal. They define normal by comparison to their peers.

For this reason, concerns about gynecomastia, even an obsession over gynecomastia, can be attributed at least in part to an increasing emphasis on male appearance. This has caused men to obsess over their appearance in ways that they perhaps would not have in the past. A passing curiosity about minor gynecomastia would cause many men today to go to their doctors requesting surgical removal. Physiologic gynecomastia in a male adolescent is nearly always reversible, as long as it does not have another contributing cause, therefore it is not medically necessary for men in this situation to undergo surgical removal.

This obsession with male appearance has led many men to resort to anabolic steroids to improve their appearance. This is an important subject in the gynecomastia discussion because androgenic compounds can lead to gynecomastia when testosterone is aromatized into estrogen, which can happen in conditions of excess free testosterone. Indeed, many men undergoing gynecomastia surgeries are men who have gynecomastia as a result of anabolic steroid use.

Related to this discussion is that of the sexual effects of gynecomastia. Gynecomastia can be associated with decreased libido in men, either because of the depression that comes along with some cases of gynecomastia or because the underlying cause of gynecomastia is also causing sexual complaints. This picture is complicated by the reality that many psychological medications can cause gynecomastia on their own and some can also cause sexual side effects, so it is not always easy to determine what the precise cause of the sexual complaints is.

Finally, gynecomastia can be treated in a number of ways. Although many people believe that the only treatment is surgery, surgery is actually not indicated in many cases, particularly when the gynecomastia is reversible. The medical provider may recommend waiting to see if the gynecomastia reverses when the inciting trigger is removed. Indeed, treating gynecomastia may be as simple as removing the trigger.

Gynecomastia, therefore, is a subject that is complex enough to write several books about, yet still approachable to the reader. Whatever your reason for reading, we hope that you gained the knowledge that you were looking for on this loaded subjected. We thank you for reading this book.